THE *Skinny*
STEAMER

RECIPE BOOK

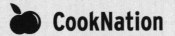

THE SKINNY STEAMER RECIPE BOOK

Delicious Healthy, Low Calorie, Steam Cooking Recipes Under 300, 400 & 500 Calories

Copyright © Bell & Mackenzie Publishing Limited 2014

ISBN 978-1-909855-67-0

A CIP catalogue record of this book is available from the British Library

DISCLAIMER

Some recipes may contain nuts or traces of nuts. Those suffering from any allergies associated with nuts should avoid any recipes containing nuts or nut based oils.

This information is provided and sold with the knowledge that the publisher and author do not offer any legal or other professional advice.

In the case of a need for any such expertise consult with the appropriate professional.

This book does not contain all information available on the subject, and other sources of recipes are available.

This book has not been created to be specific to any individual's requirements.

Every effort has been made to make this book as accurate as possible. However, there may be typographical and or content errors. Therefore, this book should serve only as a general guide and not as the ultimate source of subject information.

This book contains information that might be dated and is intended only to educate and entertain.

The author and publisher shall have no liability or responsibility to any person or entity regarding any loss or damage incurred, or alleged to have incurred, directly or indirectly, by the information contained in this book.

CONTENTS

INTRODUCTION 7

VEGETABLE SIDES 13

Simple Mexican Corn 14
Garlic Butter & Chive Corn 15
Lime & Ginger Baby Carrots 16
Honeyed Carrots & Hazelnuts 17
Lemon Oil Asparagus 18
Basil Zucchini 19
Mangetout With Pine Nuts & Mint 20
Salad Potatoes & Dijon Vinaigrette 21
Purple Sprouting Broccoli & Anchovies 22
Steamed Savoy With Bacon 23
Cumin & Turmeric Cauliflower 24
Crushed Butternut Squash 25

VEGETARIAN MEALS 27

Spiced Saffron Lentils 28
Curried Dhal 29
Lime & Coconut Lentils 30
Sweet Potato Split Peas 31
Subzi Dalcha 32
Bulgar Wheat Warm Tabbouleh 33
Savoury Spiced Steamed Rice 34
Pomegranate & Mint Quinoa 35

SEAFOOD 37

Steamed Thai Fish Fillets 38
Cantonese Fish & Coriander Rice 39

Steamed Salmon & Watercress Rice ... 40

Cod With Rosemary Tomatoes ... 41

Steamed Garlic Prawns ... 42

Shrimp & Pineapple Rice ... 43

Piri Piri Prawns & Couscous ... 44

Lime Squid Salad ... 45

Oyster Sauce Fish & Broccolini ... 46

Balsamic Tuna Steak & Rice ... 47

Anchovy & Chilli Linguine ... 48

Steamed Scallop Salad ... 49

POULTRY

51

Dressed Yogurt Chicken Breasts ... 52

Lemongrass & Ginger Chicken ... 53

Honey Chicken With Savoury Lentils ... 54

Steamed Chicken & Lemon Spinach ... 55

Chicken With Tomato & Basil Sauce ... 56

Fruit Salsa Chicken & Rice ... 57

Sliced Chicken & Chickpea Salad ... 58

Honey Chicken Kebabs ... 59

Pesto Penne Chicken ... 60

Spiced Chicken & Rice ... 61

Chicken Gyoza ... 62

MEAT

63

Chinese Ground Beef ... 64

Steamed Beef & Basil Meatballs ... 65

Bratwurst & Steamed Cabbage ... 66

Lean Quarter Pounder ... 67

Steamed Oyster Sauce Steak ... 68

Smoked Sausage Dinner ... 69

Lamb & Mint Couscous ... 70

Steamed Citrus Pork ... 71

Pork & Prawn Dumplings ... 72

EGGS, OMELETTES & FRITTATAS

	73
Cheese & Chive Omelette	74
Eggs & Ham Snack	75
Spanish Omelette	76
Chinese Eggs	77
Spinach & Feta Frittata	78
Hardboiled Eggs & Prawns	79

FRUIT

	81
Steamed Bananas	82
Steamed Cinnamon & Sultana Apples	83
Chinese Pears	84
Pineapple & Banana Rafts	85
Steamed Ginger Peaches	86

OTHER COOKNATION TITLES

	87

INTRODUCTION

The healthy and nutritious nature of steaming makes it ideal for anyone looking to maintain a low calorie diet.

Steaming is a wonderful method of cooking which is versatile, simple and healthy. The popularity of steam cooking has seen a resurgence in recent years as demand for more nutritious and reduced fat meals has increased. The nature of steaming means that foods retain more of their valuable vitamins and nutrients when compared to boiling and because cooking oils are not required, fat content is less.

Steaming works by boiling water continuously which in turn vaporizes into steam. It is this steam and heat that cooks the food keeping it moist and tender. The food in a steamer makes no contact with the boiling water. The steam circulates around the steaming tiers evenly cooking your food to perfection.

While there are numerous new electrical steamers on the market today, the method of cooking by steam is an ancient one. The Chinese have been using steam to cook for more than 3000 years and even today it is still widely used on a daily basis. In the west, steaming is more often used to cook vegetables and fish however there are many rice, meat and poultry dishes that are perfect for the steamer. Our recipes include a fantastic mix of vegetable, seafood and meat dishes.

The healthy and nutritious nature of steaming makes it ideal for anyone looking to maintain a low calorie diet. If you are following a calorie controlled diet or are keen to maintain and manage your weight our skinny steaming recipes all fall below 300, 400 and 500 calories per portion. Each delicious recipe makes two servings and have been tried, tasted & tested in both a stove-top and electric tiered steamer.

STEAMERS

There are different options to choose when steaming your food. Below is a brief description of each.

ELECTRIC STEAMERS

These are the most popular steamers and are very reasonably priced. The benefit of using an electric steamer is that it heats up the water and begins to steam almost immediately so is a quicker method of cooking. It also means your hob/stove top is free (and clean!). All electric steamers come with a timer so your food will not overcook meaning you can leave the device to do its job while you get on with other things. There are different sizes of appliances ranging from single tier to two or three tiers to suit larger families. Most have see-through plastic tiers so you can watch your food cooking and are generally dishwasher friendly.

STOVE-STOP STEAMERS

These work on the same principle as electric steamers. A large pan forms the base in which water is brought to the boil. There are a further two or three tiers that sit on top of this pan where food is placed to steam. Generally you cannot see food in these tiers as they are stainless steel although the top tier will usually have a see-through glass lid.

BAMBOO STEAMERS

Popular in Asian cooking, bamboo steamers are predominantly used over boiling water in a wok but can also be used with a pan. These can be stacked to provide two or three tiers. The advantage of bamboo steamers is that they are cheap to buy and the bamboo absorbs moisture that might normally condense on the underside of the steamer lid.

The disadvantage to this type of steaming is that they are difficult to clean, cannot be placed in the dishwasher and the bamboo may absorb and retain the flavour of the food you are cooking.

As with any kitchen appliance, convenience, suitability, reliability, performance and price are all factors in deciding which one works best for you.

STEAMING TIPS

- Always ensure there is enough water in your pan/steamer to last for the length of the steaming process and remember to top up if necessary.
- Always try to use the freshest possible ingredients when steaming. Fruit and veg that are damaged or not completely fresh can have a tainted taste when steamed. The steaming process accentuates the taste of the food.
- Use lean meat and fish. Lean products require less cooking time.
- All food should ideally be of a similar size to ensure even cooking.
- When using tiers, place the food that will take longest to cook on the bottom tier and the food that takes less time on the upper tiers.
- Make sure there is adequate space around the food in the steamer compartment to allow steam to circulate and cook evenly.
- Defrost frozen meat, fish and poultry before steaming.
- When using the stove-top method of steaming, ensure that the bottom layer does not make contact with the water otherwise the food will boil and not steam.
- Ensure the lid of your steamer fits correctly to prevent steam from escaping.
- Any foods that are likely to drip when cooking should always be placed on the bottom tier of your steamer to avoid tainting other foods.
- Steaming times in the recipes should be treated as a guide only. Always check that your food is cooked through before serving.

OUR SKINNY RECIPES

All our recipes are simple to make, easy to follow and all fall below 300, 400 or 500 calories per serving. Many use low calorie and low fat alternatives to everyday products. We would encourage you to add these to your shopping basket each week and make a point of paying attention to food labelling whenever you can - some low fat products can be very high in sugar so watch out! Try switching to some of the following everyday items to keep calories and fat lower and be sure to take note of our kitchen essentials later in this chapter:

- **Fat free yogurt**
- **Skimmed or semi skimmed milk**
- **Reduced fat cheese**
- **Low fat/unsaturated 'butter' spreads**
- **Low fat crème fraiche/low fat cream**
- **Low cal cooking oil spray**
- **Low fat mayonnaise**
- **Low fat single cream**

NUTRITION

All of the recipes in this collection are balanced low calorie meals that should help keep you feeling full. It is important to balance your food between proteins, good carbs, dairy, fruit and vegetables.

Protein. Keeps you feeling full and is also essential for building body tissue. Good protein sources come from meat, fish and eggs.

Carbohydrates. Not all carbs are good and generally they are high in calories, which makes them difficult to include in a calorie limiting diet. However carbs are a good source of energy for your body as they are converted more easily into glucose (sugar) providing energy. Try to eat 'good carbs' which are high in fibre and nutrients e.g. whole fruits and veg, nuts, seeds, whole grain cereals, beans and legumes.

Dairy. Dairy products provide you with vitamins and minerals. Cheeses can be very high in calories but other products such as low fat Greek yoghurt, crème fraiche and skimmed milk are all good.

Fruit & Vegetables. Eat your five a day. There is never a better time to fill your 5 a day quota. Not only are fruit and veg very healthy, they also fill up your plate and are ideal snacks when you are feeling hungry.

CALORIE CONSCIOUS SIDE SUGGESTIONS

If you want to make any of the recipes or snacks in this book more substantial you may want to add an accompaniment to them. Here's a list of some key side vegetables, salad, noodles etc which you may find useful when working out your calories.

All calories are per 100g/3½oz. Rice and noodle measurements are cooked weights:

	Calories		Calories
Asparagus	20	Mixed salad leaves	17
Beansprouts	20	Mushrooms	22
Brussel Sprouts	42	Pak choi/bok choy	13
Butternut Squash	45	Parsnips	70
Cabbage	30	Peas	80
Carrots	41	Peppers	40
Cauliflower:	25	Potatoes	88
Celery	14	Rocket	15
Courgette/zucchini	16	Long grain rice	140
Cucumber	15	Spinach	23
Egg noodles	62	Sweet Potato	86
Green beans	31	Sweet corn	60
Leeks	61	Tomatoes	18

SKINNY TIPS

If you are following a diet or generally keeping an eye on your calorie intake, here are some tips that will help you manage the way you eat.

In today's fast moving society many of use have adopted an unhealthy habit of eating. We eat as quickly as possibly without properly giving our bodies the chance to digest and feel full. Not only is this bad for your digestive system, but our bodies begin to relate food to just fuel instead of actually enjoying what we are eating.

Some simple tips for eating which may help you on your fasting days:
• Eat. Take it slow. There is no rush.
• Chew. It sounds obvious but you should properly chew your food and swallow only when it's broken down and you have enjoyed what you have tasted.
• Wait. Before reaching for second helpings wait 5-10 minutes and let your body tell you whether you are still hungry. More often than not, the answer will be no and you will be satisfied with the meal you have had. A glass of water before each meal will help you with any cravings for more.
• Avoid alcohol when you can. Alcohol is packed with calories and will counter effect any calorific reduction you are practicing with your daily meals.
• Drink plenty of water throughout the day. It's good for you, has zero calories, and will fill you up and help stop you feeling hungry.
• Drink a glass of water before and also with your meal. Again this will help you feel fuller.
• When you are eating each meal, put your fork down between bites – it will make you eat more slowly and you'll feel fuller on less food.

- Brush your teeth immediately after your meal to discourage yourself from eating more.
- If unwanted food cravings do strike, acknowledge them, then distract yourself. Go out for a walk, phone a friend, play with the kids, or paint your nails.
- Whenever hunger hits, try waiting 15 minutes and ride out the cravings. You'll find they pass and you can move on with your day.
- Remember - feeling a bit hungry is not a bad thing. We are all so used to acting on the smallest hunger pangs that we forget what it's like to feel genuinely hungry. Learn to 'own' your hunger and take control of how you deal with it.
- Get moving. Increased activity will complement your weight loss efforts. Think about what you are doing each day: choose the stairs instead of the lift, walk to the shops instead of driving. Making small changes will not only help you burn calories but will make you feel healthier and more in control of your weight loss.

ABOUT COOKNATION

CookNation is the leading publisher of innovative and practical recipe books for the modern, health-conscious cook.

CookNation titles bring together delicious, easy and practical recipes with their unique approach, making cooking for diets and healthy eating fast, simple and fun.

With a range of #1 best-selling titles - from the innovative 'Skinny' calorie-counted series, to the 5:2 Diet Recipes Collection - CookNation recipe books prove that 'Diet' can still mean 'Delicious'!

Turn to the end of this book to browse all CookNation's recipe books.

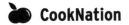 **CookNation**

COOKING GUIDE

The following times are a guide based on servings for two people. Timings may vary depending on the size of food, the space between food in the steamer and the quality of the ingredients.

Vegetables	Cooking Time (2 Portions)
Asparagus	10-15 mins
Broad beans	10-15 mins
Broccoli	10-15 mins
Shredded Cabbage	8-12 mins
Cauliflower florets	10-15 mins
Courgette	5-10 mins
Green beans	10-15 mins
Leeks	15-20 mins
Mange tout	5-10 min
Mushrooms	5-10 mins
Peas (fresh)	3-5 mins
Peas (frozen)	10-12 mins
Peppers	10-15 mins
Spinach	4-6 mins
Sprouts	15-20 mins
Sweet corn	4-6 mins
Sweet corn (frozen)	10-12 mins
Tomatoes	10-15 mins

Root Vegetables	Cooking Time (2 Portions)
Butternut squash	20-30 mins
Carrots	15-20 mins
Celeriac	20-30 mins
New potatoes	25-30 mins
Old potatoes	25-30 mins
Whole onions	20-30 mins
Swede	30-40 mins
Sweet corn on the cob	30-35 mins

Eggs	Cooking Time (2 Portions)
Soft boiled	8-10 mins
Hard boiled	11-15 mins

Meat/Poultry	Cooking Time (2 Portions)
Chicken breast (whole boneless)	15-20 mins
Duck breast (whole boneless)	20-25 mins
Chicken drumsticks	20-25 mins
Turkey escalope	15-20 mins
Pork fillet	15-20 mins
Lamb steaks	15-20 mins
Sausages	10-15 mins

Fish/Seafood	Cooking Time (2 Portions)
Thick fillet of fish	10-15 mins
Thin fillet of fish	8-12 mins
Whole fish	15-25 mins
Mussels	5-10 mins
King prawns (raw)	8-10 mins
Scallops	4-6 mins

Rice/Pasta/ Noodles	Cooking Time (2 Portions)
Easy cook rice	30-35 mins
White long grain rice	30-35 mins
White basmati rice	30-35 mins
Bulgar wheat	25-30 mins
Couscous	5-10 mins
Ready-to-Wok Noodles	10 mins
Egg noodles	10-15 mins
Pasta	15-20 mins

Fruit	Cooking Time (2 Portions)
Pears	20-25 mins
Bananas (in skin)	12-15 mins
Apples	15-18 mins

Skinny
STEAMER
VEGETABLE SIDES

SIMPLE MEXICAN CORN

200
calories per serving

Ingredients

LIGHT LUNCH

- 2 fresh medium corn on the cob
- 1 tbsp extra virgin olive oil
- 2 tsp paprika
- 2 tsp lime juice
- Salt & pepper to taste

Method

1 Remove the silky husks from the fresh corn.

2 Place the naked cobs into the steamer on the bottom tier, cover with the lid and steam for 20-30 minutes or until the fresh corn in tender. Meanwhile combine together the olive oil, paprika & lime juice.

3 When the corn is tender remove from the steamer and brush with the spiced oil.

4 Season well and serve.

CHEFS NOTE
Substitute paprika for a little cayenne pepper is you prefer your corn spicy hot.

GARLIC BUTTER & CHIVE CORN

170 calories per serving

Ingredients

FRESH & CRUNCHY

- 2 fresh medium corn on the cob
- 25g/1oz low fat 'butter' spread
- 2 garlic cloves, crushed
- 1 tbsp freshly chopped chives
- Salt & pepper to taste

Method

1 Remove the silky husks from the fresh corn.

2 Place the naked cobs into the steamer on the bottom tier, cover with the lid and steam for 10 minutes.

3 Add the butter, garlic and chives to a ramekin dish, cover tightly with foil and place on a tier above the steaming corn.

4 Cover the steamer back over with the lid and continue to steam the corn for a further

5 10-20 minutes or until the corn is cooked through.

6 When the corn is tender remove from the steamer and brush evenly with the garlic butter. Season well and serve.

CHEFS NOTE
Use a low fat olive 'butter' spread.

LIME & GINGER BABY CARROTS

80 calories per serving

Ingredients

USE FRESH LIMES

- 200g/7oz fresh baby carrots
- 25g/1oz low fat 'butter' spread
- 1 tsp freshly grated ginger
- 1 garlic clove, crushed
- 2 tsp lime juice
- Large pinch of salt
- Salt & pepper to taste

Method

1 Scrub the carrots and place into the bottom tier of the steamer. Cover with the lid and steam for 10 minutes.

2 Add the butter, ginger, garlic, lime juice & salt to a ramekin dish, cover tightly with foil and place on a tier above the steaming carrots.

3 Cover the steamer back over with the lid and continue to steam the carrots for a further 10-15 minutes, or until the carrots are cooked through and tender.

4 Place in a bowl, pour over the melted butter and combine really well until the carrots are evenly coated.

5 Season and serve.

CHEFS NOTE
Try adding some lime zest to the carrots too.

HONEYED CARROTS & HAZELNUTS

120
calories per
serving

Ingredients

SWEET & STICKY

- 200g/7oz fresh baby carrots
- 1 bunch spring onions/scallions
- 1 tbsp clear honey
- 1 tbsp hazelnuts, chopped
- Salt & pepper to taste

Method

1 Scrub the carrots and halve lengthways, along with the spring onions.

2 Place into the bottom tier of the steamer, cover with the lid and steam for 10 minutes.

3 Add the honey to a ramekin dish, cover tightly with foil and place on a tier above the steaming carrots to gently soften.

4 Cover the steamer back over with the lid and continue to steam the carrots for a further 10 minutes, or until the carrots and spring onions are cooked through and tender.

5 Place in a bowl, pour over the softened honey and combine well.

6 Sprinkle with the chopped hazelnuts and serve.

CHEFS NOTE
Try using chopped almonds in place of hazelnuts.

LEMON OIL ASPARAGUS

90
calories per
serving

Ingredients

QUICK TO MAKE!

- 200g/7oz asparagus tips
- 1 tbsp lemon juice
- 1 tsp olive oil
- Salt & pepper to taste

Method

1 Place the asparagus tips on the bottom tier of the steamer, cover with the lid and steam for 10-12 minutes or until tender.

2 Mix the olive oil and juice together. Place the asparagus in a bowl, pour over the lemon oil, combine well, season and serve.

CHEFS NOTE
A little grated Parmesan cheese makes a good addition to this simple side dish.

BASIL ZUCCHINI

90 calories per serving

Ingredients

FRESH & FAST

- 3 medium courgettes, sliced
- 1 tbsp lemon juice
- 1 tbsp olive oil
- 2 tbsp freshly chopped basil
- Salt & pepper to taste

Method

1 Place the sliced courgettes on the bottom tier of the steamer, cover with the lid and steam for 5-7 minutes or until tender.

2 Mix the lemon juice & olive oil together.

3 Place the steamed courgettes slices in a bowl and pour over the lemon oil. Combine well, sprinkle with fresh basil, season and serve.

CHEFS NOTE
Try cutting the courgettes lengthways into long thick slices rather than into discs.

MANGETOUT WITH PINE NUTS & MINT

140 calories per serving

Ingredients

NUTTY & LIGHT

- 200g/7oz mangetout
- 1 tbsp olive oil
- 1 tbsp fresh mint, finely chopped
- 1 tbsp pine nuts
- Salt & pepper to taste

Method

1 Place the mangetout on the bottom tier of the steamer, cover with the lid and steam for 5-7 minutes or until tender.

2 Meanwhile, very gently toast the pine nuts in a dry frying pan for a couple of minutes until browned (be careful not to burn them).

3 Mix the olive oil and mint together.

4 Place the mangetout in a bowl and pour over the minted oil. Combine well, sprinkle with the toasted pine nuts, season and serve.

CHEFS NOTE
Sugarsnap peas will work equally well for recipe.

SALAD POTATOES & DIJON VINAIGRETTE

245 calories per serving

Ingredients

GREAT FOR PICNICS

- 500g/1lb 2oz small salad potatoes
- 1 tbsp lemon juice
- ½ garlic clove, crushed
- 1 tbsp Dijon mustard
- 1 tbsp olive oil
- 1 bunch spring onions/scallions, chopped
- Salt & pepper to taste

Method

1 Slice the potatoes in half and place in the steamer on the bottom tier. Cover with the lid and steam for 15-20 minutes or until the potatoes are tender.

2 Meanwhile combine the lemon juice, garlic, mustard and oil together in a bowl with a good pinch of salt to make a basic vinaigrette dressing.

3 When the potatoes are tender add to the dressing and combine well.

4 Season and serve with the spring onions scattered over the top.

CHEFS NOTE
Charlotte potatoes are a good choice for this recipe.

PURPLE SPROUTING BROCCOLI & ANCHOVIES

110
calories per serving

Ingredients

→ **BEST IN SPRING**

- 200g/7oz purple sprouting broccoli
- 1 tbsp olive oil
- 2 anchovy fillets or 1 tsp anchovy paste
- 1 garlic clove, crushed
- Salt & pepper to taste

Method

1 Place the broccoli into the bottom tier of the steamer. Add the oil, anchovy fillets and garlic to a ramekin dish. Cover tightly with foil and place on a tier above the broccoli.

2 Cover the steamer with the lid and steam for 8-10 minutes or until the broccoli is tender.

3 Give the anchovies and oil a good stir to break up the fillets. Place the broccoli in a bowl, pour over the warmed anchovy oil. Combine well, season and serve.

CHEFS NOTE
Use tenderstem broccoli if you can't find purple sprouting broccoli.

STEAMED SAVOY WITH BACON

140 calories per serving

Ingredients

CHEAP TO MAKE!

- ½ savoy cabbage, shredded
- 1 tsp low fat 'butter' spread
- 4 slices lean, back bacon
- Salt & pepper to taste

Method

1 Preheat the grill to a medium heat.

2 Place the shredded cabbage into the bottom tier of the steamer. Cover with the lid and steam for 10-15 minutes or until the cabbage is tender.

3 Meanwhile grill the bacon slices for a few minutes until cooked through. Finely slice and place in a bowl.

4 Add cabbage, 'butter' and plenty of black pepper to the bacon. Combine well. Check the seasoning and serve.

CHEFS NOTE
You could also make this simple side dish using chopped Brussels sprouts.

CUMIN & TURMERIC CAULIFLOWER

70
calories per serving

Ingredients

→ **AROMATIC**

- 300g/11oz cauliflower florets
- 1 tsp each ground cumin & turmeric
- 2 tbsp fat free Greek yogurt
- 2 tsp lemon juice
- Salt & pepper to taste

Method

1 Combine the cauliflower florets, cumin, turmeric & a pinch of salt together, making sure the dry spices evenly coat the florets.

2 Place the spiced florets into the bottom tier of the steamer. Cover with the lid and steam for 10-12 minutes or until tender. Remove from the steamer and leave to cool for a minute.

3 Mix together the yogurt and lemon juice in a bowl. Add the cauliflower florets. Combine well, season and serve.

CHEFS NOTE
Leaving the cauliflower to cool for a minute discourages the excess steam from spoiling/splitting the yogurt dressing.

CRUSHED BUTTERNUT SQUASH

190 calories per serving

Ingredients

CREAMY →

- ½ butternut squash, peeled & deseeded
- Pinch of salt
- ½ tsp each chopped fresh rosemary & thyme
- 1 tsp olive oil
- 1 tbsp low fat cream
- Salt & pepper to taste

Method

1 Cube the butternut squash and combine with the salt, rosemary, thyme and olive oil.

2 Place in the bottom tier of the steamer. Cover with the lid and steam for 20-30 minutes or until the squash is tender.

3 Remove the squash from the steamer, lightly crush with the back of a fork, add the single cream and combine well. Season and serve.

CHEFS NOTE
Feel free to use dried herbs if that's all you have to hand.

Skinny
STEAMER
VEGETARIAN MEALS

SPICED SAFFRON LENTILS

260
calories per
serving

Ingredients

- 125g/4oz lentils
- 370ml/1½ cups hot vegetable stock
- 1 garlic clove, crushed
- ½ tsp each ground coriander/cilantro, cumin & turmeric

- Large pinch of saffron threads
- 1 tbsp lemon juice
- ½ tsp each brown sugar & salt
- Salt & pepper to taste

Method

1 Combine all the ingredients in a steam-proof glass bowl.

2 Place the bowl in the bottom tier of the steamer. Cover the steamer with the lid and steam for 50-60 minutes or until the lentils are tender and cooked through. (Stir once or twice during cooking and add additional stock if required). Top up the water level on your steamer as required.

3 Season and serve.

CHEFS NOTE
This is tasty just as it comes or you can serve with your choice of chopped fresh herbs.

CURRIED DHAL

330 calories per serving

Ingredients

- 125g/4oz lentils
- 370ml/1½ cups hot vegetable stock
- 2 garlic cloves, crushed
- 200g/7oz chopped fresh tomatoes
- 200g/7oz carrots, cut into batons
- 1 tbsp medium curry powder
- ½ tsp each brown sugar & salt
- 1 tbsp mango chutney
- 1 onion, chopped
- Salt & pepper to taste

Method

1 Combine all the ingredients, except the mango chutney & chopped onion, in a steam-proof glass bowl.

2 Place the bowl in the bottom tier of the steamer. Cover the steamer with the lid and steam for 50-60 minutes or until the lentils are tender and cooked through. (Stir once or twice during cooking and add additional stock if required). Top up the water level on your steamer as required.

3 Combine together the mango chutney and chopped onion.

4 Season and serve the cooked dhal with a dollop of the mango chutney and chopped onion on the side.

CHEFS NOTE
Use hot curry powder if you prefer.

LIME & COCONUT LENTILS

290 calories per serving

Ingredients

- 125g/4oz lentils
- 370ml/1½ cups hot vegetable stock
- 1 onion, chopped
- 2 garlic cloves, crushed
- 1 tbsp medium curry powder
- ½ tsp each brown sugar & salt

- 1 tbsp lime juice
- Zest of ½ lime
- 1 tbsp coconut cream
- 1 tbsp freshly chopped coriander/cilantro
- Salt & pepper to taste

Method

1 Combine all the ingredients, except the coconut cream and chopped coriander, in a steam-proof glass bowl.

2 Place the bowl in the bottom tier of the steamer. Cover the steamer with the lid and steam for 50-60 minutes or until the lentils are tender and cooked through. (Stir once or twice during cooking and add additional stock if required). Top up the water level on your steamer as required.

3 When the lentils are tender, stir through the coconut cream, sprinkle with chopped coriander and serve.

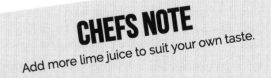

CHEFS NOTE
Add more lime juice to suit your own taste.

SWEET POTATO SPLIT PEAS

370 calories per serving

Ingredients

- 125g/4oz yellow split peas
- 370ml/1½ cups hot vegetable stock
- 1 onion, chopped
- 250g/9oz sweet potato, peeled & diced
- 1 garlic clove, crushed
- 1 tsp each garam masala & turmeric
- ½ tsp cayenne pepper
- 75g/3oz spinach
- Salt & pepper to taste

Method

1 Combine all the ingredients, except the spinach, in a steam-proof glass bowl.

2 Place the bowl in the bottom tier of the steamer. Cover the steamer with the lid and steam for 70-80 minutes or until the split peas are tender and cooked through. (Stir once or twice during cooking and add additional stock if required). Top up the water level on your steamer as required.

3 When the peas are ready, stir through the spinach for a few seconds and serve.

CHEFS NOTE

Combine the spinach with the peas for a little longer if you prefer it wilted.

SUBZI DALCHA

320
calories per serving

Ingredients

- 125g/4oz yellow split peas
- 370ml/1½ cups hot vegetable stock
- 300g/11oz mixed vegetables
- 2 garlic cloves, crushed
- 2 tsp turmeric
- 1 tsp cumin

- ½ tsp ground ginger & chilli powder
- 3 curry leaves
- 2 tbsp fat free Greek Yogurt
- ½ - 1 red chilli, deseeded & finely chopped
- Salt & pepper to taste

Method

1 Combine all the ingredients, except the yogurt and chopped chilli, in a steam-proof glass bowl.

2 Place the bowl in the bottom tier of the steamer. Cover the steamer with the lid and steam for 70-80 minutes or until the split peas are tender and cooked through. (Stir once or twice during cooking and add additional stock if required). Top up the water level on your steamer as required.

3 When the peas are ready, remove the curry leaves and serve with a dollop of yogurt in the centre of the dish sprinkled with fresh chopped chillies.

CHEFS NOTE

Use any combination of mixed vegetables you prefer – even a frozen prepared mix will work well.

BULGAR WHEAT WARM TABBOULEH

140 calories per serving

Ingredients

- 125g/4oz bulgar wheat
- 250ml/1 cup hot vegetable stock
- ½ red onion, chopped
- Pinch of ground cinnamon
- 1 tbsp lemon juice
- 2 fresh tomatoes chopped
- Large bunch of freshly chopped herbs
- Lemon wedges to serve
- Salt & pepper to taste

Method

1 Combine all the ingredients, except the chopped herbs and lemon wedges, in a steam-proof glass bowl.

2 Place the bowl in the bottom tier of the steamer. Cover the steamer with the lid and steam for 30-40 minutes or until the bulgar wheat is tender and cooked through. (Stir once during cooking and add additional stock if required).

3 When the wheat is ready, fluff it up with a fork and leave to cool for a few minutes. Quickly fold through the chopped herbs and serve with lemon wedges.

CHEFS NOTE
Equal quantities of mint, basil and flat leaf parsley make a good combination of fresh herbs for this dish.

SAVOURY SPICED STEAMED RICE

400 calories per serving

Ingredients

- 150g/5oz basmati rice
- 370ml/1½ cups hot vegetable stock
- 1 onion, chopped
- 1 garlic clove, crushed
- 75g/3oz peas
- 75g/3oz sliced mushrooms
- 1 red pepper, deseeded & chopped
- 1 tbsp medium curry powder
- 2 fresh tomatoes, chopped
- Salt & pepper to taste

Method

1 Combine all the ingredients in a steam-proof glass bowl.

2 Place the bowl in the bottom tier of the steamer. Cover the steamer with the lid and cook for 30-35 minutes or until the rice is tender. (Stir only once during cooking and add additional stock if required).

3 When the rice is ready, check the seasoning and serve.

CHEFS NOTE

Try serving with some chopped spring onions sprinkled over the top.

POMEGRANATE & MINT QUINOA

290 calories per serving

Ingredients

- 100g/3½oz quinoa
- 370ml/1½ cups hot vegetable stock
- 1 tsp lemon juice
- 1 bunch mint, finely chopped
- Seeds from 2 whole pomegranates
- Salt & pepper to taste

Method

1 Combine the quinoa and stock in a steam-proof glass bowl.

2 Place the bowl in the bottom tier of the steamer. Cover the steamer with the lid and cook for 30-35 minutes or until the quinoa is tender and the stock has been absorbed. (Stir only once during cooking and add additional stock if required).

3 When the quinoa is ready fluff it up with a fork and toss through the lemon juice, mint and pomegranate seeds. Season and serve.

CHEFS NOTE

The easiest way to extract pomegranate seeds is to cut the fruit in half. Place face down on a chopping board and bang the back of each halve hard with a spoon.

Skinny
STEAMER
SEAFOOD

STEAMED THAI FISH FILLETS

240 calories per serving

········· *Ingredients* ·········

- 2 firm white fish fillets, each weighing 175g/6oz
- ½ tsp cayenne pepper
- 1 tsp freshly grated ginger
- 1 garlic clove, crushed
- Zest of 1 lime

- 2 tbsp lime juice
- 2 tbsp soy sauce
- ½ tsp brown sugar
- 2 small Chinese cabbages (pak choi/bokchoy), shredded
- Salt & pepper to taste

········· *Method* ·········

1 Mix the cayenne pepper, ginger, garlic, zest, lime juice, soy sauce & sugar together to make a marinade in a large bowl. Add the shredded cabbage and combine really well.

2 Place the fish fillets side by side on a large piece of tin foil. Season the fish and scatter the shredded cabbage & marinade on top.

3 Fold the foil into a loose parcel around the fish leaving enough room for the steam to circulate freely around the top and sides of the fillets.

4 Place in the bottom tier of the steamer. Cover with the lid and steam for 10-15 minutes or until the fish is cooked through and the cabbage is tender.

6 Arrange on the plate, season and serve.

CHEFS NOTE
Add fresh sliced chillies and spring onions as a garnish if you want extra spice and crunch.

CANTONESE FISH & CORIANDER RICE

390 calories per serving

Ingredients

- 100g/3½oz long grain rice
- 250ml/1 cup vegetable stock
- 2 firm white fish fillets, each weighing 150g/5oz
- ½ tsp coarse sea salt
- 1 tsp freshly grated ginger
- 1 tsp sesame oil

- 2 tbsp soy sauce
- Large bunch spring onions/scallions sliced lengthways
- 4 tbsp freshly chopped coriander/ cilantro
- Salt & pepper to taste

Method

1 Combine the rice & stock in a steam-proof glass bowl and place in the second tier of the steamer. Cover the steamer with the lid and steam for 20 minutes.

2 Meanwhile rub the sea salt into the fish fillets. Mix together the oil & ginger and brush evenly over the top of the fish.

3 Place the fish side by side on a large piece of tin foil. Fold the foil into a loose parcel leaving enough room for the steam to circulate freely around the top and sides of the fillets.

4 Put the foil parcel in the bottom tier of the steamer. Cover with the lid and steam for 10-15 minutes or until the fish is cooked through and the rice is tender. (Stir the rice only once during cooking and add additional stock if required.)

5 When the rice is cooked, fluff it up with a fork and fold through the chopped coriander.

6 Arrange the fillets on a plate with the rice on the side. Spoon the soy sauce over the fish and scatter with spring onions. Serve immediately.

STEAMED SALMON & WATERCRESS RICE

400 calories per serving

Ingredients

- 100g/3½oz long grain rice
- 250ml/1 cup boiling water
- Large pinch of salt
- 2 boneless salmon fillets, each weighing 150g/5oz

- 2 tsp lemon juice
- 2 tbsp white wine
- Large handful fresh watercress, chopped
- Salt & pepper to taste

Method

1 Combine the rice, water & salt in a steam-proof glass bowl and place in the second tier of the steamer. Cover the steamer with the lid and steam for 20 minutes.

2 Place the fish fillets side by side on a large piece of tin foil, season well and pour over the lemon juice & white wine. Fold the foil into a loose parcel leaving enough room for the steam to circulate freely around the top and sides of the fillets.

3 Place the foil parcel in the bottom tier of the steamer. Cover with the lid and steam for 10-15 minutes or until the fish is cooked through and the rice is tender. (Stir the rice only once during cooking and add additional water if required.)

5 When the rice is cooked fluff it up with a fork and quickly combine with the chopped watercress.

6 Arrange the fillets on a plate with the rice on the side. Spoon any juices from the foil over the fish and serve.

CHEFS NOTE
Chopped chives are also good added to the cooked rice.

COD WITH ROSEMARY TOMATOES

280 calories per serving

Ingredients

- 2 firm white fish fillets, each weighing 175g/6oz
- 1 garlic clove, crushed
- 4 vine ripened tomatoes, sliced
- 1 tsp freshly chopped rosemary
- ½ tsp brown sugar
- 150g/5oz rocket
- 1 tbsp low fat mayonnaise
- Salt & pepper to taste

Method

1 Place the garlic, sliced tomatoes, rosemary and sugar in a small bowl and gently combine.

2 Place the fish fillets side by side on a large piece of tin foil. Season the fish and lay the dressed tomatoes over the top of the fillets.

3 Fold the foil into a loose parcel leaving enough room for the steam to circulate freely around the top and sides of the fillets.

4 Place in the bottom tier of the steamer. Cover with the lid and steam for 15-18 minutes or until the fish is cooked through and the tomatoes are tender.

5 Arrange the fish and tomatoes on a plate, with the rocket on the side along with a dollop of low fat mayo.

CHEFS NOTE
Dried rosemary is also fine to use with this recipe.

STEAMED GARLIC PRAWNS

490 calories per serving

Ingredients

- 100g/3½oz long grain rice
- 250ml/1 cup boiling water
- Large pinch of salt
- 400g/14oz raw, shelled king prawns/ jumbo shrimp

- 3 garlic cloves, crushed
- 1 tbsp olive oil
- Lemon Wedges to serve
- 2 tbsp chopped flat leaf parsley
- Salt & pepper to taste

Method

1 Combine the rice, water & salt in a steam-proof glass bowl and place in the second tier of the steamer. Cover the steamer with the lid and steam for 25 minutes.

2 Combine the prawns, garlic & oil together and place on a large piece of tin foil. Season well and fold the foil into a loose parcel leaving enough room for the steam to circulate freely around the top and sides of the prawns.

3 Place the foil parcel in the bottom tier of the steamer. Cover with the lid and steam for 5-10 minutes or until the prawns are cooked through and the rice is tender. (Stir the rice only once during cooking and add additional water if required.)

4 When the rice is cooked, fluff it up with a fork and place in shallow bowls. Pile the cooked prawns on top, sprinkle over the chopped parsley and serve with lemon wedges.

CHEFS NOTE
Fresh peas tossed though the rice are great with this simple supper.

SHRIMP & PINEAPPLE RICE

465
calories per serving

Ingredients

- 100g/3½oz long grain rice
- 250ml/1 cup hot vegetable stock
- 300g/11oz raw, shelled king prawns/ jumbo shrimp
- 150g/5oz peas
- 125g/4oz pineapple chunks, chopped
- 1 tbsp soy sauce
- Salt & pepper to taste

Method

1 Combine the rice & stock in a steam-proof glass bowl and place in the second tier of the steamer. Cover the steamer with the lid and steam for 25 minutes.

2 Place the prawns, peas & pineapple in the bottom tier of the steamer. Cover with the lid and steam for 5-10 minutes or until the prawns are cooked through and the rice is tender. (Stir the rice only once during cooking and add additional stock if required.)

3 Toss everything, including the soy sauce, together. Check the seasoning and serve.

CHEFS NOTE

If you are using frozen peas they may need a little longer in the steamer, make sure they are tender before serving.

PIRI PIRI PRAWNS & COUSCOUS

400 calories per serving

Ingredients

- 2 red chillies, deseeded
- 2 garlic cloves
- 1 tbsp olive oil
- 1 tbsp lemon juice
- 1 tbsp white wine vinegar
- ½ tsp salt
- 300g/11oz raw, shelled king prawns/ jumbo shrimp
- 100g/3½oz couscous
- 180ml/¾ cup hot vegetable stock
- 50g/2oz rocket
- Salt & pepper to taste

Method

1 Add the chillies, garlic, olive oil, lemon juice, vinegar & salt to a food processor and whizz into a paste. Remove the blade, add the prawns and combine well.

2 Put the couscous & stock in a steam-proof glass bowl and stir once. Place the chilli-covered prawns on top of the couscous and put the bowl in the bottom tier of the steamer. Cover the steamer with the lid and steam for 5-10 minutes or until the prawns are cooked through.

3 Use a fork to fluff up the couscous and toss everything well. Serve with the rocket piled on top.

CHEFS NOTE
Adjust the chilli to suit your own taste in this spicy dish.

LIME SQUID SALAD

220 calories per serving

Ingredients

- 300g/11oz prepared squid, cut into rings
- 1 red chilli, deseeded & finely chopped
- 2 garlic cloves, crushed
- 1 tbsp fish sauce
- 1 tbsp lime juice
- 1 tbsp soy sauce
- ½ tsp brown sugar
- 1 romaine lettuce shredded
- 150g/5oz cherry tomatoes, halved
- Salt & pepper to taste

Method

1 Season the squid.

2 Add the chopped chilli, garlic, fish sauce, lime juice, soy sauce & sugar to a ramekin dish. Cover tightly with foil and place on bottom tier of the steamer along with the squid rings.

3 Cover the steamer with the lid and steam for 3-6 minutes or until the squid is cooked through.

4 Serve the squid on a bed of shredded lettuce and tomatoes with the hot lime dressing poured over the top.

CHEFS NOTE
You could toss the squid in the dressing first before adding to the salad.

OYSTER SAUCE FISH & BROCCOLINI

SERVES 2

290 calories per serving

Ingredients

- 2 firm white fish fillets, each weighing 175g/6oz
- 1 tsp freshly grated ginger
- 1 garlic clove, crushed
- 2 tbsp oyster sauce
- 2 tbsp soy sauce
- 250g/9oz tenderstem broccoli
- Salt & pepper to taste

Method

1 Mix together the ginger, garlic, oyster & soy sauces in a bowl to form a marinade.

2 Place the fish fillets side by side on a large piece of tin foil and brush with a little of the marinade.

3 Add the broccoli to the remainder of the marinade in the bowl and combine well. Tip this over the fish and fold the foil into a loose parcel leaving enough room for the steam to circulate freely around the top and sides of the fillets and broccoli.

4 Place in the bottom tier of the steamer. Cover with the lid and steam for 10-15 minutes or until the fish is cooked through and the broccoli is tender.

5 Arrange on the plate, season and serve.

CHEFS NOTE
Broccolini refers to any variety of young tenderstem broccoli.

BALSAMIC TUNA STEAK & RICE

470 calories per serving

Ingredients

- 100g/3½oz long grain rice
- 250ml/1 cup hot vegetable stock
- 2 fresh tuna steaks, each weighing 150g/5oz
- 3 tbsp balsamic vinegar
- 1 garlic clove, crushed
- 2 tbsp soy sauce
- Salt & pepper to taste

Method

1 Combine the rice & stock in a steam-proof glass bowl and place in the second tier of the steamer. Cover the steamer with the lid and steam for 20 minutes.

2 Season the tuna. Mix together the balsamic vinegar, garlic & soy sauce in a small ramekin dish. Cover with a piece of foil and place on the bottom tier of the steamer alongside the seasoned tuna steaks.

3 Cover with the lid and steam for a further 10-12 minutes or until the tuna is cooked through and the rice is tender.

4 Serve the tuna steaks on a bed of rice with the balsamic sauce poured over the top.

CHEFS NOTE
Serve with some finely shredded spring onions/scallions.

ANCHOVY & CHILLI LINGUINE

Ingredients

- 150g/5oz linguine, snapped in half
- Large pinch of salt
- 5 anchovy fillets, drained
- 2 tbsp olive oil
- 1 tsp dried crushed chillies
- 2 garlic cloves, peeled
- Lemon wedges to serve
- Salt & pepper to taste

Method

1 Place the pasta in a steam-proof glass bowl, cover with boiling water and add a pinch of salt. Place in the bottom tier of the steamer, cover with the lid and steam for 5 minutes.

2 Meanwhile add the anchovy fillets, oil & crushed chillies to a ramekin dish and place alongside the bowl with the pasta in it. Add the garlic cloves to the tier and continue to steam for 10-15 minutes or until the pasta is cooked through and the garlic is tender.

3 After this time drain the pasta. Crush the steamed garlic and combine well with the warm anchovy fillets; making sure the anchovies are broken up really well.

5 Toss the garlic anchovy oil through the pasta. Season and serve with lemon wedges.

CHEFS NOTE
You could also sauté a slice red onion whilst the pasta is cooking and toss this through the sauce with the oil.

STEAMED SCALLOP SALAD

170 calories per serving

Ingredients

- 8 shelled, cleaned scallops
- 2 tbsp soy sauce
- 2 tsp clear honey
- ½ tsp crushed chilli flakes
- 1 tbsp lime juice
- 1 tsp freshly grated ginger
- 200g/7oz mixed salad leaves
- Salt & pepper to taste

Method

1 Combine together the soy sauce, honey, chilli flakes, lime juice & ginger to make a dressing. Quickly toss the scallops with the dressing until well covered (reserving any remaining dressing).

2 Place the scallops in the bottom tier of the steamer. Cover with the lid and steam for approximately 4-5 minutes or until just cooked through.

3 Serve on a bed of mixed salad leaves with any remaining dressing drizzled over the top.

CHEFS NOTE
Use the freshest scallops you can get your hands on.

Skinny
STEAMER
POULTRY

DRESSED YOGURT CHICKEN BREASTS

340 calories per serving

Ingredients

- 2 chicken breasts, each weighing 150g/5oz
- 1 tsp dried thyme
- 1 lemon, thinly sliced
- 2 garlic cloves, peeled

- 250g/9oz asparagus tips
- 2 tbsp fat free Greek yogurt
- 1 tsp Dijon mustard
- 1 tsp clear honey
- Salt & pepper to taste

Method

1 Season the chicken breasts, sprinkle with thyme and place on the bottom tier of the steamer. Place the garlic cloves in there too and then cover the chicken breasts with the lemon slices.

2 Cover with the lid and leave to steam for 10 minutes. After this time place the asparagus tips in the second tier and steam for 10 minutes longer or until the chicken is cooked through and the asparagus is tender.

3 Remove the steamed garlic and crush. Gently combine this with the yogurt, mustard & honey to make a dressing.

4 Arrange the chicken and asparagus on the plate and serve with the yogurt dressing poured over the chicken breast.

CHEFS NOTE
Include some of the lemon slices from the steamer on the plate if you wish.

LEMONGRASS & GINGER CHICKEN

480 calories per serving

Ingredients

- 1 tsp fish sauce
- 1 garlic clove, crushed
- 1 tsp soy sauce
- 1 red chilli, deseeded & finely chopped
- 1 tsp freshly grated ginger
- 1 tbsp clear honey
- 1 lemongrass stalk, finely chopped

- 2 chicken breasts, each weighing 150g/5oz
- 125g/5oz peas
- 100g/3½oz long grain rice
- 250ml/1 cup boiling water
- Large pinch of salt
- Salt & pepper to taste

Method

1 Combine together the fish sauce, garlic, soy, chilli, ginger, honey and chopped lemongrass to make a marinade.

2 Use your hands to rub the marinade into the chicken breast and put to one side to allow the flavour to develop.

3 Meanwhile combine the rice, water & salt in a steam-proof glass bowl and place in the second tier of the steamer. Cover the steamer with the lid and steam for 10 minutes.

4 Add the marinated chicken breasts to the bottom tier of the steamer and add the peas to the steam-proof bowl with the rice.

5 Cover the steamer and leave to cook for a further 20 minutes or until the chicken is cooked through and the rice tender.

6 Cut the chicken into thick slices and use a fork to fluff up the pea rice. Serve in shallow bowls with the chicken slices on top of the rice.

CHEFS NOTE
Try spinach or sugar snaps peas in the rice if you like.

HONEY CHICKEN WITH SAVOURY LENTILS

440 calories per serving

Ingredients

- 100g/3½oz lentils
- 250ml/1 cup hot vegetable stock
- 2 chicken breasts, each weighing 150g/5oz

- 1 tsp clear honey
- 1 tsp soy sauce
- 2 tbsp freshly chopped basil
- Salt & pepper to taste

Method

1 Combine the lentils and stock in a steam-proof glass bowl and place on the second tier of the steamer. Cover the steamer with the lid and cook for 40 minutes.

2 Brush the chicken breasts with the honey and soy sauce, place in the bottom tier of the steamer, cover and cook for a further 20 minutes or until the chicken is cooked through and the lentils are tender (stir the lentils once or twice during cooking and add additional stock if required).

3 Cut the chicken breasts into thick slices, and serve with the lentils on the side sprinkled with fresh basil.

CHEFS NOTE
Red lentils are best for this recipe.

54

STEAMED CHICKEN & LEMON SPINACH

320 calories per serving

Ingredients

- 2 chicken breasts, each weighing 150g/5oz
- 2 garlic cloves, crushed
- 1 tsp olive oil
- 2 courgettes, thinly sliced lengthways
- ½ onion, finely chopped
- 150g/5oz spinach
- 2 tsp lemon juice
- Salt & pepper to taste

Method

1 Place the chicken breasts side by side on a large piece of tin foil. Mix together the garlic & olive oil and brush over the chicken fillets.

2 Lay the courgettes slices and chopped onions on top of the chicken and fold the foil into a loose parcel leaving enough room for the steam to circulate freely around the top and sides of the chicken breasts and courgettes.

3 Place in the bottom tier of the steamer. Cover with the lid and steam for 20 minutes or until the chicken is cooked through. Add the spinach to the second tier of the steamer, cover and steam for a further 2-3 minutes or until the spinach has wilted.

4 Transfer the spinach to a bowl, toss with the lemon juice and a good pinch of salt.

5 Remove the chicken and courgette parcel from the steamer and serve on plates with the spinach on the side.

CHEFS NOTE

Try garnishing the spinach with sesame seeds and a little extra olive oil.

CHICKEN WITH TOMATO & BASIL SAUCE

310 calories per serving

Ingredients

- 2 chicken breasts, each weighing 150g/5oz
- 1 garlic clove, crushed
- 4 tbsp tomato ketchup

- Large bunch of fresh basil
- 300g/11oz cherry tomatoes
- 150g/5oz watercress
- Salt & pepper to taste

Method

1 Season the chicken. Add the garlic clove, ketchup, basil and tomatoes to a food processor and pulse for a few seconds to make a chunky sauce. Put the sauce in a steam-proof dish and cover with a piece of foil.

2 Place the chicken breasts in the bottom tier and the sauce dish in the second tier of the steamer. Cover with the lid and steam for 20 minutes or until the chicken is cooked through.

3 Plate up the chicken, pour over the tomato sauce and serve with the watercress on the side.

CHEFS NOTE
Fresh oregano makes a good alternative to basil.

FRUIT SALSA CHICKEN & RICE

440 calories per serving

Ingredients

- 100g/3½oz long grain rice
- 250ml/1 cup boiling water
- Large pinch of salt
- 2 chicken breasts, each weighing 125g/4oz
- 1 small bunch fresh coriander/cilantro
- 1 small bunch spring onions/scallions
- 1 tbsp lime juice
- 200g/7oz tinned pineapple chunks
- Salt & pepper to taste

Method

1 Combine the rice, water and salt in a steam-proof glass bowl and place in the second tier of the steamer. Cover the steamer with the lid and steam for 15 minutes.

2 Meanwhile season the chicken. Add the fresh coriander, spring onions, lime juice & pineapple to a food processor and pulse for a few seconds to make a chunky fruit salsa. Put the salsa in a small steam-proof dish and cover with a piece of foil.

3 Place the chicken and salsa dish in the bottom tier of the steamer. Cover with the lid and steam for 20 minutes or until the chicken is cooked through.

4 Serve the chicken on a bed of rice with the hot salsa poured over the top.

CHEFS NOTE
Add a little fresh chopped chilli to the salsa if you like.

SLICED CHICKEN & CHICKPEA SALAD

440
calories per serving

Ingredients

- 2 chicken breasts, each weighing 125g/4oz
- 4 tbsp dry cider
- 2 tsp wholegrain mustard
- 1 tbsp honey

- 200g/7oz tinned chickpeas, drained
- 200g/7oz rocket
- 2 tsp lemon juice
- 4 tbsp low fat cream
- Salt & pepper to taste

Method

1 Season the chicken. Combine together the cider, mustard & honey in a ramekin dish and cover with a piece of foil.

2 Place the chicken and ramekin dish in the bottom tier of the steamer. Cover with the lid and steam for 20 minutes or until the chicken is cooked through.

3 Toss the chickpeas, rocket and lemon juice together. Slice the chicken thickly and lay on top of the rocket and chickpeas. Stir the cream through the warm honey in the ramekin dish and pour over the chicken salad.

CHEFS NOTE
Use English mustard if you want the salad dressing to have more of a 'bite'.

HONEY CHICKEN KEBABS

380 calories per serving

Ingredients

- 300g/11oz chicken breasts, cubed
- 1 garlic clove, crushed
- 2 tbsp soy sauce
- 1 tbsp clear honey
- 1 tbsp olive oil
- 200g/7oz cherry tomatoes
- 1 tbsp freshly chopped flat leaf parsley
- Salt & pepper to taste
- Wooden kebab sticks

Method

1 Place the cubed chicken, garlic, soy sauce, honey, olive oil & cherry tomatoes in a bowl and combine really well.

2 Place the honey-covered chicken and cherry tomatoes onto wooden skewers in turn to make 4-6 kebabs.

3 Place the kebabs on the bottom tier of the steamer, cover with the lid and leave to steam for 10-15 minutes or until the chicken is cooked through.

4 Sprinkle with the chopped parsley, season and serve.

CHEFS NOTE
You could use cubed peppers and whole button mushrooms on the skewers too.

PESTO PENNE CHICKEN

498
calories per
serving

Ingredients

- 1 garlic clove, crushed
- 1 tbsp lemon juice
- 1 tsp dried basil
- 150g/5oz penne

- 2 chicken breasts, each weighting 125g/4oz
- 2 tbsp green pesto sauce
- Salt & pepper to taste

Method

1 Combine together the garlic, lemon juice & basil and use this to brush on to the chicken breasts. Place the chicken on the bottom tier of the steamer and cook for 10 minutes.

2 Place the pasta in a steam-proof glass bowl, cover with boiling water and add a pinch of salt. Place in the second tier of the steamer, cover with the lid and steam for a further 15 minutes or until the pasta is tender and the chicken is cooked through.

3 Remove the chicken and cut each breast into thick slices. Drain the pasta and combine well with the pesto sauce.

4 Serve the pesto penne in shallow bowls with the chicken breast arranged on top.

CHEFS NOTE
If you prefer you could shred the chicken and stir this through the pesto penne.

SPICED CHICKEN & RICE

420 calories per serving

Ingredients

- 100g/3½oz long grain rice
- 250ml/1 cup boiling water
- Large pinch of salt
- Large pinch of saffron threads
- 2 tbsp chopped sultanas
- 2 chicken breasts, each weighing 125g/4oz
- ½ tsp each ground coriander/cilantro, cumin, turmeric and cayenne pepper
- 2 tbsp mango chutney
- Salt & pepper to taste

Method

1 Combine the rice, water, salt & saffron in a steam-proof glass bowl and place in the second tier of the steamer. Cover the steamer with the lid and steam for 10 minutes.

2 Meanwhile mix together the dried spices and coat the chicken breasts in these. Place the chicken in the bottom tier of the steamer and add the chopped sultanas to the rice. Cover with the lid and steam for 20-25 minutes or until the chicken is cooked through and the rice is tender.

3 Slice the chicken thickly on a bed of rice with a tablespoon of mango chutney on the side.

CHEFS NOTE
If you don't have any saffron, cook the rice in chicken stock instead.

CHICKEN GYOZA

385
calories per
serving

Ingredients

- 250g/9oz chicken mince/ground chicken
- Handful of finely shredded cabbage
- 2 garlic cloves, crushed
- ½ tsp each ground ginger & crushed chilli
- 1 tbsp oyster sauce
- 1 tbsp soy sauce
- ½ tsp each salt & brown sugar
- 10-12 ready-made gyoza skins
- 2 tbsp sweet chilli dipping sauce
- Salt & pepper to taste

Method

1 Place all the ingredients, except the dumpling wrapper & sweet chilli sauce, into a food processor. Pulse a couple of times until everything is well combined.

2 Lay out the gyoza skins and place about 2 teaspoons of the chicken mixture into the centre of each skin. Wet the edges with a little water, fold over and pinch the newly closed edge to make a little parcel.

3 Place the dumplings in the bottom tier of the steamer. Cover with the lid and steam for 10-12 minutes or until the dumplings are cooked through.

4 Serve with the sweet chilli dipping sauce.

CHEFS NOTE
You could also use minced prawns or pork for this simple Japanese dumpling recipe. You can find gyoza skins in Asian stores.

Skinny
STEAMER
MEAT

CHINESE GROUND BEEF

490 calories per serving

Ingredients

- 100g/3½oz long grain rice
- 250ml/1 cup boiling water
- Large pinch of salt
- 250g/9oz lean beef mince/ground beef
- 1 tsp grated ginger
- 2 tsp soy sauce
- 1 egg
- 1 garlic clove, crushed
- 1 tbsp hoisin sauce
- Bunch spring onions/scallions, chopped
- Salt & pepper to taste

Method

1 Combine the rice, water & salt in a steam-proof glass bowl and place in the second tier of the steamer. Cover the steamer with the lid and steam for 10 minutes.

2 Meanwhile use your hands to mix together the mince, ginger, soy sauce, egg & garlic and form into two flat meat patties about 2cm/1 inch thick. Brush with hoisin sauce and place in the bottom tier of the steamer.

3 Cover the steamer with the lid and steam for a further 15-20 minutes or until the rice is tender and the beef is cooked through.

4 Arrange on a plate, sprinkle with spring onions and serve.

CHEFS NOTE
You could use oyster sauce in place of hoisin.

STEAMED BEEF & BASIL MEATBALLS

490 calories per serving

Ingredients

- 100g/3½oz long grain rice
- 250ml/1 cup boiling water
- Large pinch of salt
- 250g/9oz lean beef mince/ground beef
- 1 tbsp Worcestershire sauce/A1 steak sauce
- 1 egg
- 1 bunch fresh basil, chopped (reserve a little for garnish)
- 1 garlic clove, crushed
- Salt & pepper to taste

Method

1 Combine the rice, water & salt in a steam-proof glass bowl and place in the second tier of the steamer. Cover the steamer with the lid and steam for 10 minutes.

2 Meanwhile use your hands to mix together the mince, Worcestershire sauce, egg, fresh basil & garlic. Form into 8-10 small meatballs and place in the bottom tier of the steamer.

3 Cover the steamer with the lid and steam for a further 15-20 minutes or until the rice is tender and the meatballs are cooked through.

4 Serve in a shallow bowl with the meatballs piled on top, sprinkled with the reserved fresh basil.

CHEFS NOTE
You may like to serve with a simple tomato sauce or gravy.

BRATWURST & STEAMED CABBAGE

495 calories per serving

Ingredients

- 250g/9oz bratwurst sausage
- 1 tbsp low fat 'butter' spread
- 1 garlic clove, crushed

- 1 green pointed cabbage, shredded
- 1 tbsp grated Parmesan cheese
- Salt & pepper to taste

Method

1 Place the bratwurst in bottom tier of the steamer

2 Add the butter & garlic to a ramekin dish and cover tightly with foil. Place this and the shredded cabbage in the second tier of the steamer.

3 Cover the steamer with the lid and cook for 10-15 minutes or until the sausages are cooked through and the cabbage is tender.

4 Remove the sausages and cut into thick slices diagonally. Toss the garlic butter with the cabbage and arrange in a shallow bowl. Place the sausage on top and sprinkle with Parmesan cheese and lots of black pepper.

CHEFS NOTE
Use any type of sausage you prefer for this traditional German supper.

LEAN QUARTER POUNDER

460 calories per serving

Ingredients

- 250g/9oz lean beef mince/ground beef
- 1 garlic clove, crushed
- 1 egg, beaten
- 1 tsp Worcestershire sauce/A1 steak sauce
- 1 tsp Dijon Mustard

- 2 slices low fat cheddar cheese
- 1 vine ripened tomato, sliced
- 1 baby gem lettuce, shredded
- 2 regular wholemeal burger rolls
- Salt & pepper to taste

Method

1 Place the beef, garlic, egg, Worcestershire sauce and mustard into a bowl. Mix really well and form into two burger patties.

2 Place the burgers in the bottom tier of the steamer, cover with the lid and steam for 10-15 minutes or until the burgers are cooked through.

3 Place the cheese on top of the burgers and steam for a couple of minutes (if you want the cheese melted).

4 To serve; assemble the burgers in the rolls with the shredded lettuce & sliced tomatoes.

CHEFS NOTE

Try using a plastic burger maker. They are cheap to buy and vastly improve the texture of the burger.

SERVES 2

STEAMED OYSTER SAUCE STEAK

340 calories per serving

Ingredients

- 3 tbsp oyster sauce
- ½ tsp each salt & brown sugar
- 1 tsp soy sauce
- 1 garlic clove, crushed
- 250g/9oz trimmed sirloin steak, cut into strips

- 2 pak choi/bok choi, quartered
- 2 carrots cut into batons
- 1 red pepper, deseeded & finely sliced
- 1 bunch spring onions/scallions sliced lengthways
- Salt & pepper to taste

Method

1 In a steam-proof bowl combine together the oyster sauce, salt, sugar, soy sauce and garlic to form a marinade. Add the sliced steak to the bowl, mix well and place in the bottom tier of the steamer.

2 Put the pak choi, carrots and peppers in the second tier of the steamer and cook for 10-15 minutes or until the steak is cooked to your liking and the vegetables are tender.

3 Combine the vegetables and steak together and serve in a shallow bowl sprinkled with the spring onions.

CHEFS NOTE
You could serve this with fine egg noodles or beansprouts too.

68

SMOKED SAUSAGE DINNER

490 calories per serving

Ingredients

- 150g/5oz penne
- 200g/7oz reduced fat smoked sausage
- 1 tsp Worcestershire sauce/A1 steak sauce
- 250ml/1 cup tomato passata/sauce
- 1 tbsp tomato puree/paste
- ½ tsp each salt & brown sugar
- 1 garlic clove, peeled
- Salt & pepper to taste

Method

1 Place the pasta in a steam-proof glass bowl, cover with boiling water and add a pinch of salt. Place in the bottom tier of the steamer along with the smoked sausage.

2 Add the Worcestershire sauce, passata, puree, salt & sugar to a separate steam-proof bowl and combine well. Cover tightly with foil and put in the second tier of the steamer. Place the garlic clove beside it.

3 Cover the steamer with the lid and cook for 15 minutes or until the pasta is tender and the sausage is cooked through.

4 Crush the garlic and add to the tomato sauce. Drain the pasta & thickly slice the sausages. Combine everything together really well, check the sauce seasoning and serve immediately.

CHEFS NOTE

You may need to alter the balance of sugar and salt a little in this simple tomato sauce.

LAMB & MINT COUSCOUS

470
calories per serving

Ingredients

- 2 lean lamb steaks, each weighing 125g/4oz
- 1 garlic clove, crushed
- 1 tsp olive oil
- 2 tbsp freshly chopped mint
- 100g/3½oz couscous
- 180ml/¾ cup hot vegetable stock
- Salt & pepper to taste

Method

1 Place the lamb steaks side by side on a large piece of foil and brush with the garlic and olive oil.

2 Fold the foil into a loose parcel leaving enough room for the steam to circulate freely around the top and sides of the lamb. Place the lamb in the bottom tier of the steamer, cover with the lid and cook for 10 minutes.

3 After this time put the couscous & stock in a steam-proof glass bowl and stir once. Place in the second tier of the steamer. Cover with the lid and steam for a further 5-10 minutes or until the lamb is cooked through.

4 Use a fork to fluff up the couscous and toss the chopped mint through it.

5 Serve the lamb steaks with the minted couscous on the side. Season and serve.

CHEFS NOTE
Serve with lemon wedges.

STEAMED CITRUS PORK

395 calories per serving

Ingredients

- 2 pork loin steaks, each weighing 150g/5oz
- 2 tbsp orange juice
- 1 tbsp freshly chopped coriander/cilantro
- 200g/7oz carrots, cut into batons
- 1 tsp clear honey
- 2 tsp lemon juice
- Salt & pepper to taste

Method

1 Place the pork loins side by side on a large piece of foil. Season well and pour over the orange juice and chopped coriander.

2 Fold the foil into a loose parcel leaving enough room for the steam to circulate freely around the top and sides of the pork steaks.

3 Place the carrot batons in a bowl and combine with the honey. Place the foil parcels in the bottom tier of the steamer and the carrots in the second tier.

4 Cover with the lid and steam for 18-25 minutes or until the pork is cooked through and the carrots are tender.

CHEFS NOTE

This is also good served with some roasted gnocchi.

PORK & PRAWN DUMPLINGS

360 calories per serving

Ingredients

- 125g/4oz lean mince pork/ground pork
- 125g/4oz raw prawns/shrimp
- 1 tbsp soy sauce
- 1 tbsp fish sauce
- ½ tsp ground ginger
- 1 tsp cornflour/cornstarch
- 10-12 wonton dumpling wrappers
- 2 tbsp plum sauce
- Salt & pepper to taste

Method

1 Place all the ingredients, except the dumpling wrappers & plum sauce, into a food processor. Pulse a couple of times until everything is really well combined.

2 Lay out the wonton wrappers and place about 2 teaspoons of the pork mixture into the centre of each paper. Gather the sides up and pinch the top to form a closed parcel.

3 Place the dumplings in the bottom tier of the steamer. Cover with the lid and steam for 10-12 minutes or until the dumplings are cooked through.

4 Serve with the plum dipping sauce.

CHEFS NOTE

Ready-made wonton dumpling wrappers are widely available in larger supermarkets or Asian stores.

Skinny
STEAMER
EGGS, OMELETTES
& FRITTATAS

CHEESE & CHIVE OMELETTE

170 calories per serving

Ingredients

USE FREE RANGE

- 4 eggs
- 50g/2oz low fat grated cheddar cheese
- 4 tbsp chopped chives
- Salt & pepper to taste

Method

1 Combine all the ingredients together.

2 Split the mixture evenly between two shallow, lightly greased, steam-proof dishes.

3 Place on the first and second tier of the steamer. Cover with the lid and steam for 8-10 minutes or until the eggs are set. Fold each omelette in half and serve.

CHEFS NOTE
Omelettes make a super easy low calorie lunch or supper.

EGGS & HAM SNACK

190
calories per
serving

Ingredients

QUICK & EASY

- 4 eggs
- 2 slices lean smoked ham, chopped
- 2 tsp sundried tomato puree
- Salt & pepper to taste

Method

1 Combine all the ingredients together.

2 Split the mixture evenly between two greased ramekin dishes.

3 Place on the bottom tier of the steamer. Cover with the lid and steam for 15-20 minutes or until the eggs are set. Eat straight out of the dishes with a fork.

CHEFS NOTE
This is a perfect lunchtime snack.

SPANISH OMELETTE

Ingredients

SPICY !

- 6 eggs
- 50g/2oz chorizo sausage, finely chopped
- 1 tsp paprika
- 1 tbsp freshly chopped flat leaf parsley
- Salt & pepper to taste

Method

1 Combine all the ingredients together.

2 Pour the mixture into a well-greased, shallow, steam-proof dish.

3 Place on the bottom tier of the steamer. Cover with the lid and steam for 8-12 minutes or until the eggs are set. Cut into thick wedges and serve.

CHEFS NOTE
This traditional thick omelette is good served with a simple green & tomato salad.

CHINESE EGGS

120
calories per
serving

Ingredients

EASTERN SPECIALITY

- 3 eggs
- 180ml/¾ cup water
- 1 tsp salt
- 1 tsp sesame oil
- 1 tsp soy sauce
- 4 spring onions/scallions sliced lengthways
- Salt & pepper to taste

Method

1 Beat the eggs together really well and pass through a sieve into a steam-proof dish. Add the water and salt and mix well.

2 Let the mixture settle for a few minutes. Cover tightly with tin foil and place into the bottom tier of the steamer.

3 Cover with the lid and steam for 20-25 minutes or until the eggs are set.

4 Garnish with a drop of sesame oil, soy sauce and the finely chopped spring onions.

CHEFS NOTE
Transfer the raw egg mixture into two small ramekin dishes before cooking if you prefer to serve each portion individually.

SPINACH & FETA FRITTATA

280
calories per
serving

Ingredients

IRON RICH

- 6 eggs
- 50g/2oz spinach, finely chopped
- 50g/2oz low fat feta cheese, crumbled
- Salt & pepper to taste

Method

1 Combine all the ingredients together.

2 Pour the mixture into a well-greased, shallow, steam-proof dish.

3 Place on the bottom tier of the steamer. Cover with the lid and steam for 8-12 minutes or until the eggs are set. Cut into thick wedges and serve.

CHEFS NOTE
You could use goat's cheese in place of feta.

HARDBOILED EGGS & PRAWNS

170 calories per serving

Ingredients

GREAT FOR SHARING

- 4 eggs
- 8 large cooked peeled king prawns/ jumbo shrimp (or steam raw prawns with the eggs for 8-10 minutes or cooked through)
- 1 tbsp low fat mayonnaise
- 1 tsp paprika
- 1 tbsp chopped dil or chives
- Salt & pepper to taste

Method

1 Place the eggs in a steamer and hard boil for 20 minutes. Plunge into a bowl of ice-cold water and, when they are cool enough, peel each egg.

2 Cut in half lengthways and carefully scoop out the yolks. Mash the yolks, mayonnaise and paprika together with a fork.

3 Load the paprika mash back into the egg halves, place a king prawn on top of each (use the mash to secure it) and sprinkle with the chopped dill.

4 Season with plenty of salt and pepper and serve.

CHEFS NOTE
This makes a great appetiser. You could increase the quantities and serve as a canapé for guests.

Skinny
STEAMER
FRUIT

STEAMED BANANAS

140 calories per serving

Ingredients

STICKY & SWEET ➡

- 2 large bananas
- 2 tsp clear honey
- 1 tbsp coconut cream

Method

1 Cut both ends off the bananas. Place in the bottom tier of the steamer and steam for 10-15 minutes or until the banana skins are blackened.

2 Drizzle with honey and serve with a dollop of coconut cream.

CHEFS NOTE
Try a little cinnamon sprinkled over the top of the bananas.

STEAMED CINNAMON & SULTANA APPLES

110 calories per serving

Ingredients

AROMATIC ➤

- 2 apples
- 2 tbsp sultanas
- 1 tsp brown sugar
- ½ tsp cinnamon
- 1 tsp lemon juice

Method

1 Mix together the sultanas, sugar and cinnamon.

2 Peel & core the apples. Brush all over with lemon juice and stuff the sultana mixture into the cored cavity.

3 Place the apples in the bottom tier of the steamer and steam for 15-25 minutes or until the apples are tender.

CHEFS NOTE
Serve with a dollop of fat free Greek yogurt.

CHINESE PEARS

180 calories per serving

Ingredients

SWEET & NUTTY

- 2 Asian pears
- 2 tbsp clear honey
- 1 tbsp chopped almonds

Method

1 Take a slice off the top of each pear to remove the stalk and take a small slice off the base of each pear so that it stands up on it's own.

2 Brush the honey all over the pears.

3 Place the pears in the bottom tier of the steamer and steam for 15-25 minutes or until the pears are tender.

4 Sprinkle with the chopped almonds and serve.

CHEFS NOTE
Any type of sweet pear will work for this recipe.

PINEAPPLE & BANANA RAFTS

120 calories per serving

Ingredients

KIDS FAVOURITE

- 1 banana, sliced
- 2 tinned pineapple rings
- 4 glace cherries, chopped
- 1 tsp brown sugar
- 2 tbsp fat free Greek yogurt

Method

1 Cut out two pieces of foil and lay a pineapple slice on each piece. Place the sliced banana on top of the rings along with the cherries and the brown sugar.

2 Fold the foil into two loose parcels making sure there is enough space around the side and top of the pineapple ring for the steam to circulate.

3 Place the parcels in the bottom tier of the steamer and steam for 15 minutes. Serve with a dollop of fat free Greek yogurt.

CHEFS NOTE
Double the pineapple rings in the rafts if you want a larger dessert.

STEAMED GINGER PEACHES

155 calories per serving

Ingredients

SIMPLE TO MAKE →

- 2 fresh peaches
- 1 tbsp brown sugar
- 2 tsp freshly grated ginger
- 2 tbsp fat free Greek yogurt

Method

1 Cut the peaches in half and remove the stone.

2 Distribute the chopped ginger evenly over the upturned peach halves and sprinkle with the brown sugar.

3 Place the peaches in the bottom tier of the steamer and steam for 20-25 minutes or until the peaches are tender. Serve with the Greek yogurt dolloped on top.

CHEFS NOTE
You could also use nectarines for this simple dessert.

Other COOKNATION TITLES

If you enjoyed 'The Skinny Steamer Recipe Book' we'd really appreciate your feedback. Reviews help others decide if this is the right book for them so a moment of your time would be appreciated.

Thank you.

You may also be interested in other '**Skinny**' titles in the CookNation series. You can find all the following great titles by searching under '**CookNation**'.

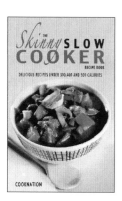

THE SKINNY SLOW COOKER RECIPE BOOK

Delicious Recipes Under 300, 400 And 500 Calories.

Paperback / eBook

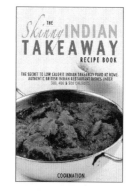

THE SKINNY INDIAN TAKEAWAY RECIPE BOOK

Authentic British Indian Restaurant Dishes Under 300, 400 And 500 Calories. The Secret To Low Calorie Indian Takeaway Food At Home.

Paperback / eBook

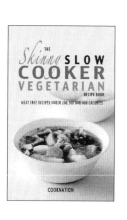

THE HEALTHY KIDS SMOOTHIE BOOK

40 Delicious Goodness In A Glass Recipes for Happy Kids.

eBook

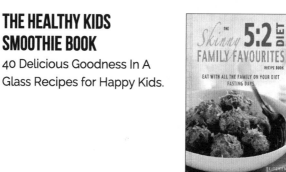

THE SKINNY 5:2 FAST DIET FAMILY FAVOURITES RECIPE BOOK

Eat With All The Family On Your Diet Fasting Days.

Paperback / eBook

THE SKINNY SLOW COOKER VEGETARIAN RECIPE BOOK

40 Delicious Recipes Under 200, 300 And 400 Calories.

Paperback / eBook

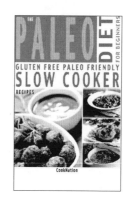

THE PALEO DIET FOR BEGINNERS SLOW COOKER RECIPE BOOK

Gluten Free, Everyday Essential Slow Cooker Paleo Recipes For Beginners.

eBook

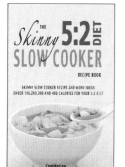

THE SKINNY 5:2 SLOW COOKER RECIPE BOOK

Skinny Slow Cooker Recipe And Menu Ideas Under 100, 200, 300 & 400 Calories For Your 5:2 Diet.

Paperback / eBook

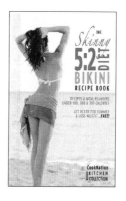

THE SKINNY 5:2 BIKINI DIET RECIPE BOOK

Recipes & Meal Planners Under 100, 200 & 300 Calories. Get Ready For Summer & Lose Weight...FAST!

Paperback / eBook

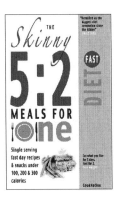

THE SKINNY 5:2 FAST DIET MEALS FOR ONE

Single Serving Fast Day Recipes & Snacks Under 100, 200 & 300 Calories.

Paperback / eBook

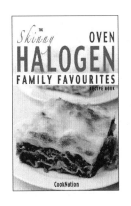

THE SKINNY HALOGEN OVEN FAMILY FAVOURITES RECIPE BOOK

Healthy, Low Calorie Family Meal-Time Halogen Oven Recipes Under 300, 400 and 500 Calories.

Paperback / eBook

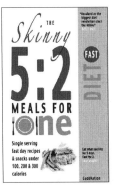

THE SKINNY 5:2 FAST DIET VEGETARIAN MEALS FOR ONE

Single Serving Fast Day Recipes & Snacks Under 100, 200 & 300 Calories.

Paperback / eBook

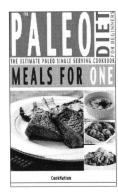

THE PALEO DIET FOR BEGINNERS MEALS FOR ONE

The Ultimate Paleo Single Serving Cookbook.

Paperback / eBook

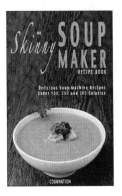

THE SKINNY SOUP MAKER RECIPE BOOK

Delicious Low Calorie, Healthy and Simple Soup Recipes Under 100, 200 and 300 Calories. Perfect For Any Diet and Weight Loss Plan.

Paperback / eBook

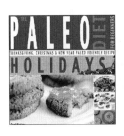

THE PALEO DIET FOR BEGINNERS HOLIDAYS

Thanksgiving, Christmas & New Year Paleo Friendly Recipes.
eBook

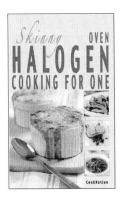

SKINNY HALOGEN OVEN COOKING FOR ONE

Single Serving, Healthy, Low Calorie Halogen Oven RecipesUnder 200, 300 and 400 Calories.

Paperback / eBook

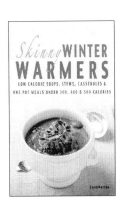

SKINNY WINTER WARMERS RECIPE BOOK

Soups, Stews, Casseroles & One Pot Meals Under 300, 400 & 500 Calories.

Paperback / eBook

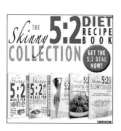

THE SKINNY 5:2 DIET RECIPE BOOK COLLECTION

All The 5:2 Fast Diet Recipes You'll Ever Need. All Under 100, 200, 300, 400 And 500 Calories.

eBook

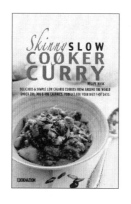

THE SKINNY SLOW COOKER CURRY RECIPE BOOK

Low Calorie Curries From Around The World.

Paperback / eBook

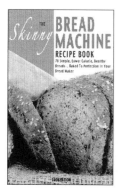

THE SKINNY BREAD MACHINE RECIPE BOOK

70 Simple, Lower Calorie, Healthy Breads...Baked To Perfection In Your Bread Maker.

Paperback / eBook

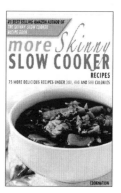

MORE SKINNY SLOW COOKER RECIPES

75 More Delicious Recipes Under 300, 400 & 500 Calories.

Paperback / eBook

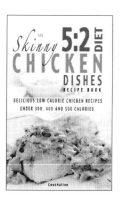

THE SKINNY 5:2 DIET CHICKEN DISHES RECIPE BOOK

Delicious Low Calorie Chicken Dishes Under 300, 400 & 500 Calories.

Paperback / eBook

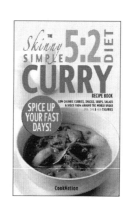

THE SKINNY 5:2 CURRY RECIPE BOOK

Spice Up Your Fast Days With Simple Low Calorie Curries, Snacks, Soups, Salads & Sides Under 200, 300 & 400 Calories.

Paperback / eBook

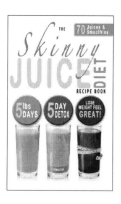

THE SKINNY JUICE DIET RECIPE BOOK

5lbs, 5 Days. The Ultimate Kick- Start Diet and Detox Plan to Lose Weight & Feel Great!

Paperback / eBook

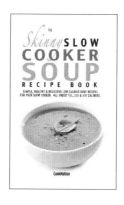

THE SKINNY SLOW COOKER SOUP RECIPE BOOK

Simple, Healthy & Delicious Low Calorie Soup Recipes For Your Slow Cooker. All Under 100, 200 & 300 Calories.

Paperback / eBook

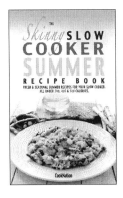

THE SKINNY SLOW COOKER SUMMER RECIPE BOOK

Fresh & Seasonal Summer Recipes For Your Slow Cooker. All Under 300, 400 And 500 Calories.

Paperback / eBook

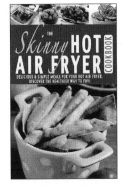

THE SKINNY HOT AIR FRYER COOKBOOK

Delicious & Simple Meals For Your Hot Air Fryer: Discover The Healthier Way To Fry.

Paperback / eBook

THE SKINNY ACTIFRY COOKBOOK

Guilt-free and Delicious ActiFry Recipe Ideas: Discover The Healthier Way to Fry!

Paperback / eBook

THE SKINNY ICE CREAM MAKER

Delicious Lower Fat, Lower Calorie Ice Cream, Frozen Yogurt & Sorbet Recipes For Your Ice Cream Maker.

Paperback / eBook

THE SKINNY 15 MINUTE MEALS RECIPE BOOK

Delicious, Nutritious & Super-Fast Meals in 15 Minutes Or Less. All Under 300, 400 & 500 Calories.

Paperback / eBook

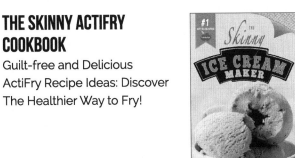

THE SKINNY SLOW COOKER COLLECTION

5 Fantastic Books of Delicious, Diet-friendly Skinny Slow Cooker Recipes: ALL Under 200, 300, 400 & 500 Calories!

eBook

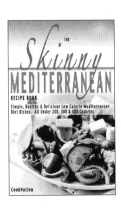

THE SKINNY MEDITERRANEAN RECIPE BOOK

Simple, Healthy & Delicious Low Calorie Mediterranean Diet Dishes. All Under 200, 300 & 400 Calories.

Paperback / eBook

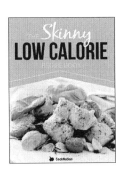

THE SKINNY LOW CALORIE RECIPE BOOK

Great Tasting, Simple & Healthy Meals Under 300, 400 & 500 Calories. Perfect For Any Calorie Controlled Diet.

Paperback / eBook

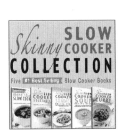

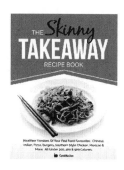

THE SKINNY TAKEAWAY RECIPE BOOK

Healthier Versions Of Your Fast Food Favourites: All Under 300, 400 & 500 Calories.

Paperback / eBook

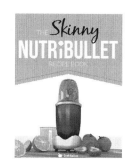

THE SKINNY NUTRIBULLET RECIPE BOOK

80+ Delicious & Nutritious Healthy Smoothie Recipes. Burn Fat, Lose Weight and Feel Great!

Paperback / eBook

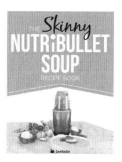

THE SKINNY NUTRIBULLET SOUP RECIPE BOOK

Delicious, Quick & Easy, Single Serving Soups & Pasta Sauces For Your Nutribullet. All Under 100, 200, 300 & 400 Calories!

Paperback / eBook

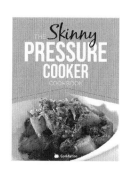

THE SKINNY PRESSURE COOKER COOKBOOK

USA ONLY
Low Calorie, Healthy & Delicious Meals, Sides & Desserts. All Under 300, 400 & 500 Calories.

Paperback / eBook

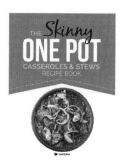

THE SKINNY ONE-POT RECIPE BOOK

Simple & Delicious, One-Pot Meals. All Under 300, 400 & 500 Calories

Paperback / eBook

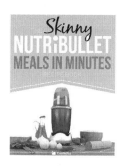

THE SKINNY NUTRIBULLET MEALS IN MINUTES RECIPE BOOK

Quick & Easy, Single Serving Suppers, Snacks, Sauces, Salad Dressings & More Using Your Nutribullet. All Under 300, 400 & 500 Calories

Paperback / eBook

CONVERSION CHART: DRY INGREDIENTS

Metric	Imperial
7g	¼ oz
15g	½ oz
20g	¾ oz
25g	1 oz
40g	1½oz
50g	2oz
60g	2½oz
75g	3oz
100g	3½oz
125g	4oz
140g	4½oz
150g	5oz
165g	5½oz
175g	6oz
200g	7oz
225g	8oz
250g	9oz
275g	10oz
300g	11oz
350g	12oz
375g	13oz
400g	14oz

Metric	Imperial
425g	15oz
450g	1lb
500g	1lb 2oz
550g	1¼lb
600g	1lb 5oz
650g	1lb 7oz
675g	1½lb
700g	1lb 9oz
750g	1lb 11oz
800g	1¾lb
900g	2lb
1kg	2¼lb
1.1kg	2½lb
1.25kg	2¾lb
1.35kg	3lb
1.5kg	3lb 6oz
1.8kg	4lb
2kg	4½lb
2.25kg	5lb
2.5kg	5½lb
2.75kg	6lb

CONVERSION CHART: LIQUID MEASURES

Metric	Imperial	US
25ml	1fl oz	
60ml	2fl oz	¼ cup
75ml	2½ fl oz	
100ml	3½fl oz	
120ml	4fl oz	½ cup
150ml	5fl oz	
175ml	6fl oz	
200ml	7fl oz	
250ml	8½ fl oz	1 cup
300ml	10½ fl oz	
360ml	12½ fl oz	
400ml	14fl oz	
450ml	15½ fl oz	
600ml	1 pint	
750ml	1¼ pint	3 cups
1 litre	1½ pints	4 cups

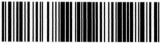

Printed in Great Britain
by Amazon.co.uk, Ltd.,
Marston Gate.